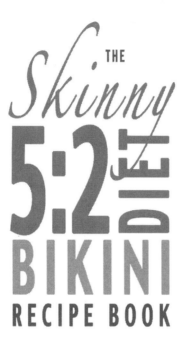

THE

Skinny

5:2 DIET

BIKINI

RECIPE BOOK

Recipes & Meal Planners Under 100, 200 & 300 Calories.

Get Ready For Summer & Lose Weight... FAST!

A Bell & Mackenzie Publication
First published in 2013 by Bell & Mackenzie Publishing

ISBN 978-0-9576447-1-7

A copy of this book is available from the British Library

Disclaimer
The information and advice in this book is intended as a
guide only. Any individual should independently seek the
advice of health professional before embarking on a diet.
Some recipes may contain nuts or traces of nuts. Those
suffering from any allergies associated with nuts should
avoid any recipes containing nuts or nut based oils.

Contents

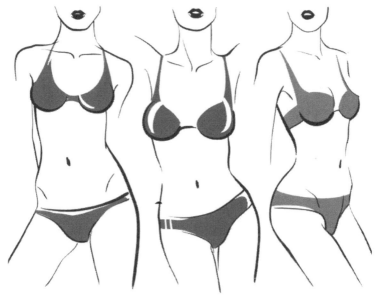

THE **5:2 DIET** *Explained*

What Is The 5:2 Diet?

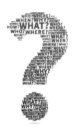

Imagine a diet where you can eat whatever you want for 5 days a week and diet for only 2. That's what the 5:2 Diet is, and it's revolutionised the way people think about dieting. With summer just around the corner, it's not too late to start getting in shape so you can be happy and confident in your swimsuit this season!

By allowing you the freedom to eat normally for MOST of the week and restrict your calorie intake for just TWO non-consecutive days a week (500 calories per day for women/600 for men), you keep yourself motivated and remove that dreaded feeling of constantly denying yourself the food you really want to eat.

It still takes willpower, but it's nowhere near as much of a grind when you know that you have tomorrow to look forward to. It's all about freedom. The ability to be flexible with the days you choose to fast makes the likelihood of you sticking to the diet for a prolonged period, or even indefinitely as a lifestyle choice, much higher than a regime that requires daily calorie restriction.

Popularised by Dr. Michael J. Mosley, the 5:2 diet plan has been adopted by both health professionals and regular people alike as a way of life which will change your relationship with dieting and weight loss. What's more, this way of eating is believed to have major health benefits which could alter your health forever!

How It Works

The concept of fasting is an ancient one and modern science is uncovering evidence that fasting can be an extremely healthy way to shed extra weight. Research has shown that it can reduce levels of IGF-1 (insulin-like growth factor 1, which leads to accelerated ageing), activate DNA repair genes, and reduce blood pressure, cholesterol and glucose levels as well as suggestions of a lower risk of heart disease and cancers.

In short, the 5:2 Diet works by restricting your body to fewer calories than it uses. Most importantly is that it does this in a way that remains healthy and is balanced by eating normally for the other 5 days of the week.

This book has been developed specifically to help you concentrate on the practice of 5:2, and to help you lose weight with our range of low calorie recipes. However if you want to find out more about the specific details of the science of the subject we would recommend Dr. Michael J. Mosley's work and, as with all diets, you should consider seeking advice from a health professional before starting.

What Will This Book Do For Me?

This book will give you a wide choice of delicious, low calorie, easy to prepare meals and snacks that will not only form the basis of your 5:2 Diet plan but also open your eyes to a new lifestyle choice. The 5:2 Diet, if followed correctly, will help you shed weight, and in the long term it can be a fantastic lifestyle choice to maintain a healthy weight while improving your overall health and immune system.

This book has been designed to help you through your 5:2 Diet journey by providing detailed menu planners, recipes and snack ideas to keep you motivated and your engine stoked during your fasting days.

What makes the 5:2 Diet so good is that it's only a part time diet. Because you can eat what you want for the other 5 days a week, you'll be much more likely to stick with it over time and enjoy the long term health and weight benefits.

Taking It Week By Week

The 5:2 diet can work for you whatever your lifestyle. Each week you should think carefully about which days are likely to be best suited to your fasting days and then stick with it. You can change your days each week or keep in a regular routine, whichever suits you best. Ideally your fasting days should be non-consecutive.

This gives you the opportunity to stay motivated by eating normally the following day, although it can be acceptable to fast for 2 days consecutively if you are feeling particularly inspired.

Of course, reducing your calorie intake for two days will take some getting used to and inevitably there will be hunger pangs to start with, but you'll be amazed at how quickly your body adapts to your new style of eating and, far from gorging the day after your fasting day, you'll find you simply enjoy the luxury of eating normally.

When Will I See Results?

By the end of your first week in most cases! Obviously everybody is different, but where someone is carrying extra weight they will normally see a reduction in the first week of embarking on the 5:2 Diet. Typically many will see a greater weight loss at the beginning, followed by a slowing down then eventually settling around a stable healthy weight.

 You could lose up to 14 lbs over a 3 month period, so start now if you want to slip into your bikini in time for summer and look and feel amazing!

How Will I Manage My Calories?

There are a number of different approaches to managing your 500 calorie intake (600 for men) on your fast days depending on your personal preferences.

We have developed 3 alternative 4-week meal planners to help you.

- **OPTION 1:** **Skip breakfast, eat lunch & dinner.**
- **OPTION 2:** **Skip lunch, eat breakfast and dinner.**
- **OPTION 3:** **Eat little and often throughout the day.**

There is much research and debate about the health benefits and risk of skipping meals, however the beauty of the 5:2 Diet is that the fasting occurs only for 2 days of the week with the remaining 5 reserved for 'normal' eating and recommended daily calorie intakes (1900-2000 for women, 2400-2500 for men). The point being that there is not a prolonged period of starving the body of calories, and eating balanced meals like those included in this book ensures that nutrition is still provided on the fasting days.

Portion Sizes

The size of the portion that you put on your plate will significantly affect your weight loss efforts. Filling your plate with over-sized portions will obviously increase your calorie intake and hamper your dieting efforts.

It's important that with all meals both on your fasting and normal eating days that you use a correct sized portion, which generally is the size of your clenched fist.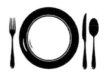

This applies to any side dishes of vegetables and carbs too. You will be surprised at how quickly you will adopt this as the 'norm' as the weeks go by and you will begin to stop over-eating.

Measurements

All recipes are for one serving but can easily be increased if you are cooking for others too. As with portion sizes, stick with the recommended measurements of ingredients. Altering these will affect your calorie intake and therefore your ultimate weight loss.

Choosing Your Fast Days

Give yourself the best possible chance of success by choosing your fast days in advance and sticking to them. As we have already said, we recommend choosing two non-consecutive fasting days so that you only have one 24 hour period at a time where you have to concentrate on limiting your calories.

It makes sense to choose your fast days sensibly based on your own particular lifestyle. For example, for many, a Friday night may involve takeaway food after a hard week at work. If this is your ritual, then avoid this as your fasting day. Similarly if you meet up with friends during the week or have a business event that is likely to involve lunch or dinner then choose an alternative day. You can alter the days each week but just remember to check your calendars and prepare in advance.

Eat, Chew, Wait

In today's fast moving society many of use have adopted an unhealthy habit of eating. We eat as quickly as possibly without properly giving our bodies the chance to digest and feel full. Not only is this bad for your digestive system, but our bodies begin to relate food to just fuel instead of actually enjoying what we are eating.

Some simple tips for eating which may help you on your fasting days:

- **Eat slowly:** there is no rush.

- **Chew:** it sounds obvious but properly chew your food and swallow only when it's broken down and you have enjoyed what you have tasted.

- **Wait before second helpings:** instead of immediately going back for more, wait for 5-10 minutes and let your body tell you whether you are still hungry. More often than not, the answer will be no and you will be satisfied with the meal you have had. A glass of water before each meal will help you with any cravings for more.

Nutrition

All of the recipes in this collection are balanced low calorie meals and snacks, which should keep you feeling full on your fasting days.

In any diet, it is important to balance your food between proteins, good carbs, dairy and fruit and vegetables.

Protein. Keeps you feeling full and is also essential for building body tissue. Good protein sources come from meat, fish and eggs.

Carbohydrates. Not all carbs are good and generally they are high in calories which makes them difficult to include in a calorie limiting diet. Carbs are a good source of energy for your body as they are converted more easily into glucose (sugar) providing energy. Try to eat 'good carbs' which are high in fibre and nutrients e.g. whole fruits and veg, nuts, seeds, whole grain cereals, beans and legumes.

Dairy. Dairy products provide you with vitamins and minerals. Cheeses can be very high in calories but other products such as low calorie Greek yoghurt, crème fraiche and skimmed milk are all good.

Fruit & Veg. Eat your five a day. There is never a better time to fill your 5 a day quota. Not only are fruit and veg very healthy, they also fill up your plate and are ideal snacks when you are feeling hungry.

Meal Planners

You'll need to find out what suits you best on your fasting days by trying out all the different options. It may suit you to skip a meal altogether or you may prefer smaller more regular eats throughout your fasting day. Either way you shouldn't take in more than 500 calories (women) /600 calories (men) per day, and this includes drinks.

The menus work on a 4 week rolling basis. So every option, whether it be leaving out lunch, breakfast or having smaller meals throughout the day, has a monthly plan of its own.

Not every meal day planner is going to work for you, and it may be unrealistic to expect you to cook twice a day if you are out at work, so feel free to substitute something else for the same calories. Likewise you may choose to prepare meals in advance so that you can stick with the planners exactly. That's the beauty of this diet, you can decide how, when and what you eat as long as you stay under 500 calories(women) or 600 calories (men) on your fasting days.

Some 5:2 Tips

Avoid too much exercise on your fasting days. Eating less is likely to make you feel a little weaker, certainly to start with, so don't put the pressure on yourself to exercise.

Avoid alcohol on your fasting days. Not only is alcohol packed with calories, it could also have a greater effect on you than usual as you haven't eaten as much.

Don't give up! Even if you find your fasting days tough to start with, stick with it. Remember you can eat what you like tomorrow without having to feel guilty.

Drink plenty of water throughout the day. Water is the best friend you have on your fasting days. It's good for you, has zero calories, and will fill you up and help stop you feeling hungry.

When you are eating each meal, put your fork down between bites – it will make you eat more slowly and you'll feel fuller on less food.

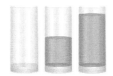 Drink a glass of water before and also with your meal. Again this will help you feel fuller.

Brush your teeth immediately after your meal to discourage yourself from eating more.

Have clear motivations. Think about what you are trying to achieve and stick with it. Remember you can eat what you want tomorrow.

If unwanted food cravings do strike, acknowledge them, then distract yourself. Go out for a walk, phone a friend, play with the kids, or paint your nails.

Whenever hunger hits, try waiting 15 minutes and ride out the cravings. You'll find they pass and you can move on with your day.

Remember - feeling hungry is not a bad thing. We are all so used to acting on the smallest hunger pangs that we forget what it's like to feel genuinely hungry. Feeling hungry for a couple of days a week is not going to harm you. Learn to 'own' your hunger and take control of how you deal with it.

If you feel you can't do it by yourself then get some support. Encourage a friend or partner to join you on the 5:2 Diet. Having someone to talk things through with can be a real help.

Get moving. Being active isn't a necessity for the 5:2 Diet to have results but as with all diets increased activity will complement your weight loss efforts. Think about what you are doing each day: choose the stairs instead of the lift, walk to the shops instead of driving. Making small changes will not only help you burn calories but will make you feel healthier and more in control of your weight loss.

Don't beat yourself up! If you have a bad day forget about it, don't feel guilty. Recognise where you went wrong and move on. Tomorrow is a new day and you can start all over again. Fast just two days a week and you'll see results. Guaranteed.

GOOD LUCK!

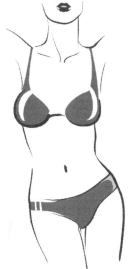

Skinny
THE
5:2 DIET
BIKINI
RECIPE BOOK

Meal Planners

Option 1: No Breakfast

Recipe Meal Planner **Week 1, Day 1** No Breakfast	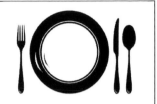
Drinks Throughout The Day: no more than 50 calories Low calorie suggestions: still & sparkling water, herbal tea, green tea, black tea, black coffee, watermelon juice	50
Lunch: Tasty Chicken Soup Recipe finder: page 66 Add 2 small breadsticks	188
Dinner: Shredded Ginger Pork Recipe finder: page 67 Add 100g/3 ½ oz green mixed salad.	214
Total Calorie Intake:	**452**

Recipe Meal Planner **Week 1, Day 2** No Breakfast	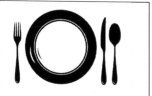
Drinks Throughout The Day: no more than 50 calories Low calorie suggestions: still & sparkling water, herbal tea, green tea, black tea, black coffee, watermelon juice	50
Lunch: Cumin Chickpea Snack Recipe finder: page 68	190
Dinner: Citrus Ground Lamb Recipe finder: page 110 Add 100g/3 /12 oz steamed pak choi	252
Total Calorie Intake:	**492**

Recipe Meal Planner

Week 2, Day 1

No Breakfast

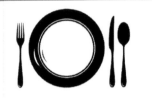

Drinks Throughout The Day: no more than 50 calories Low calorie suggestions: still & sparkling water, herbal tea, green tea, black tea, black coffee, watermelon juice	50
Lunch: Simple Sweet & Sour Drummers Recipe finder: page 111 Add 50g/2 oz sliced cucumber	221
Dinner: Tuna Potato Salad Recipe finder: page 112	229
Total Calorie Intake:	**500**

Recipe Meal Planner # Week 2, Day 2 No Breakfast	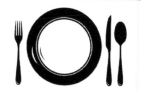

Drinks Throughout The Day: no more than 50 calories Low calorie suggestions: still & sparkling water, herbal tea, green tea, black tea, black coffee, watermelon juice	50
Lunch: Prawn & Rice Soup Recipe finder: page 69	199
Dinner: Steak & Peanut Salad Recipe finder: page 113 Add 100g/3 ½ oz beansprouts	241
Total Calorie Intake:	**490**

Recipe Meal Planner # Week 3, Day 1 No breakfast	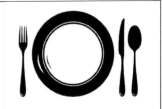

Drinks Throughout The Day: no more than 50 calories Low calorie suggestions: still & sparkling water, herbal tea, green tea, black tea, black coffee, watermelon juice	50
Lunch: Mango Melba Salad Recipe finder: page 70	199
Dinner: Red Curry Thai Chicken Recipe finder: page 114 Add 100g/3 ½ oz shirataki noodles (page 58)	246
Total Calorie Intake:	**495**

Recipe Meal Planner **Week 3, Day 2** No Breakfast	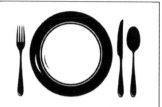
Drinks Throughout The Day: no more than 50 calories Low calorie suggestions: still & sparkling water, herbal tea, green tea, black tea, black coffee, watermelon juice	50
Lunch: Italian Beans Recipe finder: page 71	125
Dinner: Pork & Apple Medallions Recipe finder: page 115 Add 100g/ 3 ½ oz steamed spinach	299
Total Calorie Intake:	474

Recipe Meal Planner **Week 4, Day 1** No Breakfast	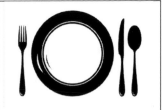

Drinks Throughout The Day: no more than 50 calories Low calorie suggestions: still & sparkling water, herbal tea, green tea, black tea, black coffee, watermelon juice	50
Lunch: Sticky Wings Recipe finder: page 72	189
Dinner: Plaice & Mixed Mushrooms Recipe finder: page 116 Add 100g/ 3 ½ oz fresh chopped tomatoes	261
Total Calorie Intake:	**500**

Recipe Meal Planner # Week 4, Day 2 No Breakfast	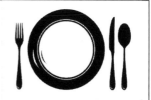

Drinks Throughout The Day: no more than 50 calories Low calorie suggestions: still & sparkling water, herbal tea, green tea, black tea, black coffee, watermelon juice	50
Lunch: Spicy Yoghurt Chicken Recipe finder: page 73 Add 100g/ 3/12 oz celery stalks	182
Dinner: The Best Mussels Recipe finder: page 117	253
Total Calorie Intake:	**485**

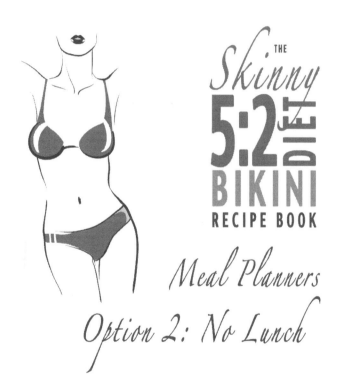

Skinny
THE
5:2 DIET
BIKINI
RECIPE BOOK

Meal Planners

Option 2: No Lunch

Recipe Meal Planner

Week 1, Day 1

No Lunch

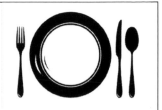

Drinks Throughout The Day: no more than 50 calories Low calorie suggestions: still & sparkling water, herbal tea, green tea, black tea, black coffee, watermelon juice	50
Breakfast: Strawberry & Banana Smoothie Recipe finder: page 53 Add ½ low fat bagel & reduced fat spread	155
Dinner: Aromatic Tuna Steaks Recipe finder: page 118 Add 100g/3 ½ oz steamed broccoli	273
Total Calorie Intake:	**498**

Recipe Meal Planner **Week 1, Day 2** No Lunch	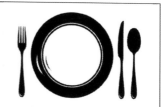
Drinks Throughout The Day: no more than 50 calories Low calorie suggestions: still & sparkling water, herbal tea, green tea, black tea, black coffee, watermelon juice	50
Breakfast: Spicy Scrambled Eggs Recipe finder: page 88 Add 2 wholewheat crackerbreads/wheat crackers	247
Dinner: Marmite Spaghetti Recipe finder: page 75	198
Total Calorie Intake:	**495**

Recipe Meal Planner

Week 2, Day 1

No Lunch

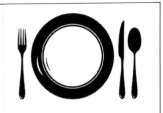

Drinks Throughout The Day: no more than 50 calories Low calorie suggestions: still & sparkling water, herbal tea, green tea, black tea, black coffee, watermelon juice	50
Breakfast: 2 weetabix & 125ml skimmed milk	175
Dinner: Spicy Lamb Fillet Recipe finder: page 119 Add 100g/3 ½ oz courgette/zucchini + 100g red cabbage	250
Total Calorie Intake:	**475**

Recipe Meal Planner

Week 2, Day 2

No Lunch

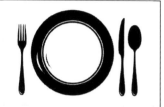

Drinks Throughout The Day: no more than 50 calories Low calorie suggestions: still & sparkling water, herbal tea, green tea, black tea, black coffee, watermelon juice	50
Breakfast: 1 small slice melon & 1 slice of Parma ham	140
Dinner: Lime & Chilli Mackerel Recipe finder: page 124 Add 50g/ 2 oz mixed salad	282
Total Calorie Intake:	**472**

Recipe Meal Planner # Week 3, Day 1 No Lunch	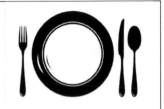

Drinks Throughout The Day: no more than 50 calories Low calorie suggestions: still & sparkling water, herbal tea, green tea, black tea, black coffee, watermelon juice	50
Breakfast: 2 slices low cal toast & reduced fat spread + 100g/ 3 ½ oz of strawberries	187
Dinner: Mexican Chicken Recipe finder: page 120 Add 50g/ 2 oz sweet corn	250
Total Calorie Intake:	**487**

Recipe Meal Planner **Week 3, Day 2** No Lunch	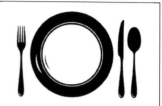
Drinks Throughout The Day: no more than 50 calories Low calorie suggestions: still & sparkling water, herbal tea, green tea, black tea, black coffee, watermelon juice	50
Breakfast: Mixed Berry Smoothie Recipe finder: page 54	100
Dinner: Pasta Carbonara Recipe finder: page 125 Add 100g/ 31/2 oz steamed spinach	317
Total Calorie Intake:	**467**

Recipe Meal Planner # Week 4, Day 1 No Lunch	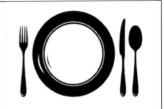

Drinks Throughout The Day: no more than 50 calories Low calorie suggestions: still & sparkling water, herbal tea, green tea, black tea, black coffee, watermelon juice	50
Breakfast: Cooked Breakfast Muffin Recipe finder: page 121	210
Dinner: Eastern Spiced Cod Steak Recipe finder: page 76 Add 100g/ 3 ½ oz pak choi + 100g/ 3 ½ oz celery	221
Total Calorie Intake:	**481**

Recipe Meal Planner

Week 4, Day 2

No Lunch

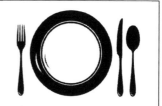

Drinks Throughout The Day: no more than 50 calories Low calorie suggestions: still & sparkling water, herbal tea, green tea, black tea, black coffee, watermelon juice	50
Breakfast: Tropical Fruit Salad Recipe finder: page 77	140
Dinner: Chicken Focaccia Recipe finder: page 122 Add 100g/3 ½ oz wild rocket salad + 100g fresh tomatoes	280
Total Calorie Intake:	**470**

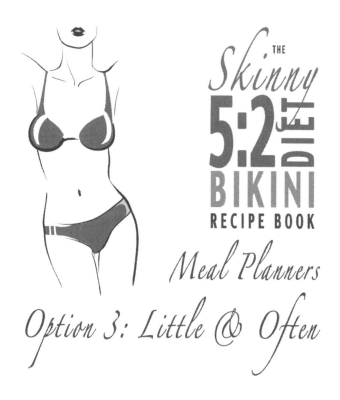

THE

Skinny

5:2 DIET

BIKINI

RECIPE BOOK

Meal Planners

Option 3: Little & Often

Recipe Meal Planner # Week 1, Day 1 Little & Often	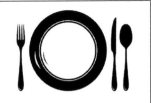

Drinks Throughout The Day: no more than 50 calories Low calorie suggestions: still & sparkling water, herbal tea, green tea, black tea, black coffee, watermelon juice	50
1 Sliced Apple & 1 Tsp Peanut Butter	100
Kiwi & Strawberry Smoothie Recipe finder: page 55	100
St Patrick's Day Soup Recipe finder: page 61	110
Italian Beans Recipe finder: page 71	125
Total Calorie Intake:	**485**

Recipe Meal Planner **Week 1, Day 2** Little & Often	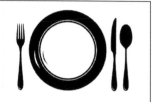

Drinks Throughout The Day: no more than 50 calories Low calorie suggestions: still & sparkling water, herbal tea, green tea, black tea, black coffee, watermelon juice	50
Perfect Egg On Toast Recipe finder: page 63	170
15g/ ½ oz Whole Almonds	83
Tuna & Capers On Oatcakes Recipe finder: page 56	100
Carrot & Celery Salad Recipe finder: page 51	97
Total Calorie Intake:	**500**

Recipe Meal Planner

Week 2, Day 1

Little & Often

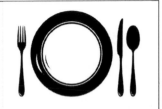

Drinks Throughout The Day: no more than 50 calories Low calorie suggestions: still & sparkling water, herbal tea, green tea, black tea, black coffee, watermelon juice	50
200g / 7 oz Watermelon	60
Grilled Chicken & Tomato Snack **Sugar Snap Peas & Sea Salt** Recipe finder: page 52 & 50	165
Pear & Roquefort Snack Salad Recipe finder: page 65	115
Boiled Egg With Soy & Sesame Oil Recipe finder: page 64	110
Total Calorie Intake:	**500**

Recipe Meal Planner # Week 2, Day 2 Little & Often	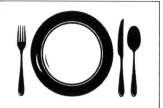
Drinks Throughout The Day: no more than 50 calories Low calorie suggestions: still & sparkling water, herbal tea, green tea, black tea, black coffee, watermelon juice	50
100g/ 3 ½ oz Strawberries	27
Mixed Berry Smoothie Recipe finder: page 54	100
Baked Brunch For 1 Recipe finder: page 85	139
Meatball Rotisserie Recipe finder: page 62	160
Total Calorie Intake:	**476**

Recipe Meal Planner # Week 3, Day 1 Little & Often	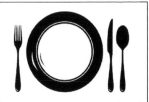

Drinks Throughout The Day: no more than 50 calories Low calorie suggestions: still & sparkling water, herbal tea, green tea, black tea, black coffee, watermelon juice	50
Homemade Salsa & 3 Tortilla Chips Recipe finder: page 48	100
Wild Mushroom Stroganoff Recipe finder: page 60	121
Tasty Chicken Soup Recipe finder: page 66	188
½ Frozen Banana	40
Total Calorie Intake:	**499**

Recipe Meal Planner **Week 3, Day 2** Little & Often	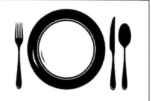

Drinks Throughout The Day: no more than 50 calories Low calorie suggestions: still & sparkling water, herbal tea, green tea, black tea, black coffee, watermelon juice	50
1 Apple	80
Baked Brunch For 1 Recipe finder: page 85	139
Chicken & Corn Skewer Recipe finder: page 78	161
100g/3 ½ oz Low Fat Baked Beans	70
Total Calorie Intake:	500

Recipe Meal Planner **Week 4, Day 1** Little & Often	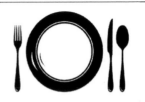	
Drinks Throughout The Day: no more than 50 calories Low calorie suggestions: still & sparkling water, herbal tea, green tea, black tea, black coffee, watermelon juice		50
Mixed Berry Smoothie Recipe finder: page 54		100
Slow Spanish Tombet Recipe finder: page 80		115
Zucchini Soup Recipe finder: page 57 Add 1 small pitta bread		172
100g / 3 ½ oz Frozen Grapes		60
Total Calorie Intake:		**497**

Recipe Meal Planner **Week 4, Day 2** Little & Often	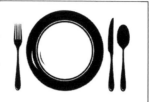

Drinks Throughout The Day: no more than 50 calories Low calorie suggestions: still & sparkling water, herbal tea, green tea, black tea, black coffee, watermelon juice	50
Tomato, Olive & Feta Salad Recipe finder: page 79	113
Shirataki Noodles & Soy Recipe finder: page 58	50
75g / 3 oz No-Fat Yoghurt With 1 Tsp Honey	90
Sheik Kebab Recipe finder: page 81	195
Total Calorie Intake:	**498**

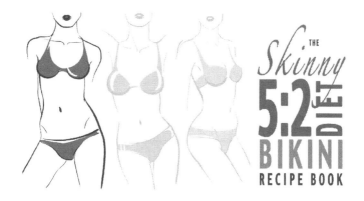

RECIPES UNDER
100 Calories

Homemade Salsa

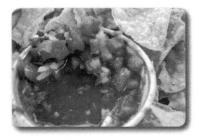

Serves: 1

Calories: 65

Ingredients:

- 125g/4oz fresh tomatoes, finely chopped

- 1/2 small onion, finely chopped

- 1 green chilli, finely chopped

- Small bunch fresh coriander (cilantro), finely chopped

- Salt, to taste

- Lime juice, to taste

Method:
Combine all ingredients together and serve.

Cucumber Salad Snack

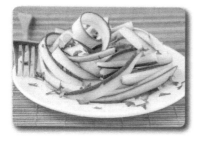

Serves: 1

Calories: 29

Ingredients:

- 75g/3oz cucumber
- 1 tsp fresh coriander/cilantro chopped
- 2 tsp lemon juice
- Pinch salt
- Pinch sugar
- 1 tsp fresh mint, chopped
- Pinch dried crushed chillies

Method:
Use a vegetable peeler to slice the cucumber into thin ribbons. Mix the lemon juice, salt, sugar and chillies together and add the cucumber ribbons. Sprinkle over the fresh herbs and serve.

Sugar Snap Peas With Sea Salt

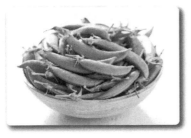

Serves: 1

Calories: 65

Ingredients:

75g/3oz sugar snap peas

1 tsp low fat spread

1 tsp crushed sea salt

1 tsp chopped fresh mint or basil

Method:

Place peas in a pan of boiling water for 1 minute, drain and then add spread & herbs into pan. When spread has melted through the peas transfer to bowl and sprinkle with sea salt.

Carrot & Celery Salad

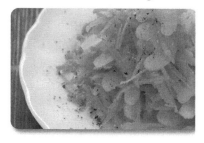

Serves: 1

Calories: 97

Ingredients:

- 2 peeled grated carrots

- 1 lemon, juiced

- 1 stalk celery, chopped

- 1 slice of tinned or fresh pineapple

- Pinch of salt

Method:
Combine all ingredients well in a bowl and serve.

Grilled Chicken & Tomato Snack

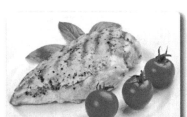

Serves: 1

Calories: 100

Ingredients:

- ½ small chicken breast
- 200g/7oz ripe cherry tomatoes

Method:
Season with plenty of salt and pepper and place your half chicken breast and cherry tomatoes (each cut in half) under the grill and leave to cook on a medium heat for 8 minutes each side (or until the chicken is thoroughly cooked). Add some fresh basil or flat leaf parsley to garnish.

Strawberry & Banana Smoothie

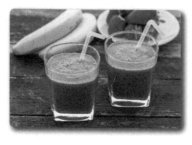

Serves: 1

Calories: 100

Ingredients:

- 125ml/ ½ cup plain fat free yoghurt
- ½ large banana

- 3 large strawberries
- Handful of ice

Method:

Add yoghurt to blender followed by other ingredients. You can use frozen or fresh fruit. Blend until smooth. Add ice to get your preferred consistency.

Mixed Berry Smoothie

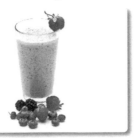

Serves: 1

Calories: 100

Ingredients:

- ½ banana
- 200g/7oz of mixed fruit berries - raspberries, blueberries, and blackberries

- 125ml/ ½ cup plain fat free yoghurt
- Handful of ice

Method:
Add yoghurt to blender followed by other ingredients. You can use frozen or fresh fruit. Blend until smooth, add ice to get your preferred consistency.

Kiwi & Strawberry Smoothie

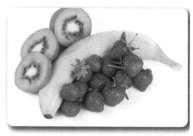

Serves: 1

Calories: 100

Ingredients:

- 1 banana
- 1 kiwi fruit
- 5 strawberries
- 1 teaspoon Agarve nectar

- Handful of ice

Method:

Add yoghurt to blender followed by other ingredients. You can use frozen or fresh fruit. Blend until smooth, add ice to get your preferred consistency.

Tuna & Capers On Oatcakes

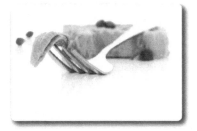

Serves: 1

Calories: 100

Ingredients:

- 40g/1 ½ oz canned tuna steak (in water)
- Squeeze of lemon juice

- 1 tsp capers, finely chopped
- 2 low calorie oat cakes

Method:
Combine tuna, capers and lemon juice together and serve on top of oatcakes.

Zucchini Soup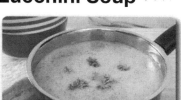

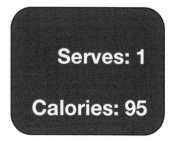

Serves: 1

Calories: 95

Ingredients:

- ¼ large potato, cubed
- 250ml/1 cup vegetable stock/broth
- ¼ head broccoli, chopped
- ¼ head cauliflower, chopped
- ½ tsp each cumin and paprika
- Salt to taste
- ¼ onion, chopped
- 1 garlic cloves, crushed
- 1 courgette, chopped
- Low cal spray

Method:

Gently sauté the onion and zucchini/courgette in the low cal cooking spray for a couple of minutes. Add all the ingredients, cover and leave to cook for 20 minutes, or until the vegetables are tender. Blend soup to required consistency.

Shirataki Noodles & Soy

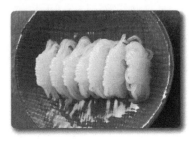

Serves: 1

Calories: 50

Ingredients:

- 100g/3 ½ oz Shirataki Noodles
- 2tsp soy sauce
- 1 tsp sesame oil
- 1 tsp fish sauce

- 1 tsp lime juice

Method:

Cook the noodles in boiling water for a few minutes. When they are tender, drain and combine with all the other ingredients.

Sometimes called 'miracle' noodles, shirataki noodles are extremely healthy low fat, low calorie noodles available widely online in the UK & USA.

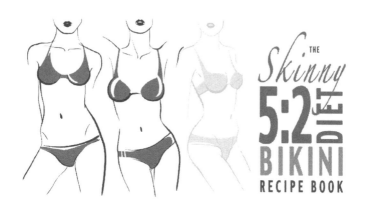

RECIPES UNDER
200 Calories

Wild Mushroom Stroganoff

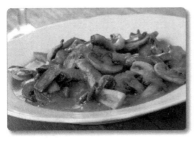

Serves: 1

Calories: 121

Ingredients:

- 140g/4 ½ oz wild mixed mushrooms sliced
- ½ onion chopped
- 1 garlic cloves crushed
- 1 tsp smoked paprika
- 60ml/ ¼ cup vegetable stock/broth

- 100g/3 ½ oz low fat condensed mushroom soup
- Small knob butter
- Bunch flat chopped leaf parsley (reserve a little for garnish)
- Salt & pepper to taste

Method:
Gently sauté the onion, garlic, mushrooms and paprika in the butter for a few minutes. Add all the other ingredients, cover and leave to gently simmer for approx. 20 minutes or until the mushrooms are lovely and tender. Season and serve.

St Patrick's Day Soup

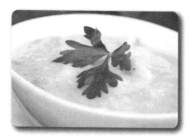

Serves: 1

Calories: 110

Ingredients:

- 1 large potato, chopped
- ½ large onion chopped
- 1 leek chopped
- Salt & pepper to taste

- 125ml/ ½ cup skimmed/low fat milk
- 250ml/ 1 cup vegetable stock/broth
- Small knob butter

Method:

Gently sauté the onion, potato and leek in the butter. Add the milk & stock and season. Leave to cooked for approx. 10-15 minutes. Make sure the potatoes are tender, and then either blend as a smooth soup or eat it rough, ready and rustic.

Meatball Rotisserie

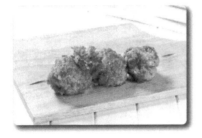

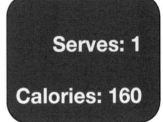

Serves: 1

Calories: 160

Ingredients:

- 100g/3 ½ oz lean minced/ground beef
- 1 small shallot, finely chopped
- ½ clove garlic, crushed
- 1 tsp ketchup
- Dash Worcestershire sauce (or chilli sauce)
- 4 ripe cherry tomatoes
- 4 small closed cup or button mushrooms
- ½ egg, beaten
- Wooden skewers
- Salt & pepper to taste
- Low cal spray

Method:

Mix together the beef, shallot, garlic, ketchup and Worcestershire sauce and, using your hands, form into 6 small meatballs. Skewer your whole mushrooms, tomatoes and meatballs in turn to make 2 little kebabs. Spray with a little low cal cooking oil and season. Place under a pre-heated medium grill and cook for approx. 10 minutes or until your meat is cooked through.

Perfect Egg On Toast

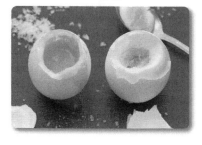

Serves: 1

Calories: 170

Ingredients:

1 small egg

1 piece low cal bread

1 scrape low cal spread

Salt & pepper to taste

Method:

Place an egg in a small pan of cold water. Cover and bring to the boil. When the water begins boiling leave for exactly 3 minutes. Meanwhile toast your bread then butter with a little low cal spread. When the egg is ready (after 3 mins of boiling) rinse in cold water and peel. Chop the egg over the toast and season.

Boiled Egg With Soy & Sesame

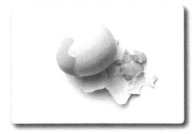

Serves: 1

Calories: 120

Ingredients:

- 1 small egg
- ½ tsp sesame oil
- ½ tsp soy sauce

- Salt & pepper to taste

Method:

Hard boil an egg for 5 minutes, allow to cool and then peel. Place the sesame oil and soy sauce in an egg cup. Dip your boiled egg in the sesame oil and soy sauce take a bite, adding salt and pepper and a dip to each bite if you prefer.

Pear & Roquefort Snack Salad

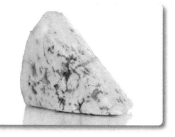

Serves: 1

Calories: 117

Ingredients:

- 15g/ ½ oz Roquefort cheese
- 2 tbsp low fat yoghurt
- 1 tsp chopped chives
- ½ ripe pear cored and cut into slices
- Pinch paprika
- Salt & pepper to taste
- 50g salad

Method:
Gently mash the cheese with the yoghurt and paprika. Season well and serve with the pear slices, and salad sprinkled with chopped chives.

Tasty Chicken Soup

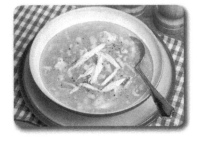

Serves: 1

Calories: 198

Ingredients:

- 7g/ ¼ oz butter
- ½ onion, chopped
- ½ stalk celery, chopped
- 1 tsp plain/ all purpose flour
- 375ml/1 ½ cups chicken stock/broth

- ½ small cooked chicken breast, chopped
- 15g/ ½ oz frozen sweet corn (optional)
- 1 tbsp flat leaf parsley, chopped
- Salt and pepper to season

Method:

Gently melt the butter in a pan with the onions and celery. When they begin to soften stir in the flour and continue cooking for a few minutes. Slowly add the stock and bring the mixture up to a good simmer. Add the sweet corn and cook for approx.10 minutes, or until everything is nice and tender. You could at this stage puree the soup to make it smooth before you add the chicken or if you prefer a more hearty texture leave as it is and throw in the chicken for a minute or two of further cooking. Season to your taste and serve with a little chopped parsley.

Shredded Ginger Pork

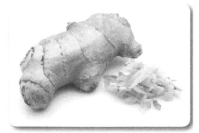

Serves: 1

Calories: 197

Ingredients:

- 1 tbsp dried Asian mushrooms, hydrated & chopped
- 75g/3 oz pork fillet
- ¼ tsp salt
- 1 tsp sunflower oil
- 1 tsp soy sauce
- 1 tsp rice vinegar
- 1 tsp fish sauce
- 1 clove garlic, crushed
- ¼ tsp brown sugar
- ¼ tsp corn flour / corn starch
- ½ tsp freshly grated ginger
- 50g/2oz fresh beansprouts
- Handful shredded cabbage
- 1 spring onion/ scallion, chopped

Method:

Mix the corn flour with a few drops of water at a time to make a paste.

Cut your pork fillet into chunks or diagonal 'chips' whichever you prefer. Mix the pork with the corn flour paste. Heat the oil in a pan and stir fry the pork. Add all the other ingredients to the pans and continue to stir-fry until everything is combined and the pork is cooked through. Garnish with the chopped spring onion and serve.

Cumin Chickpea Salad

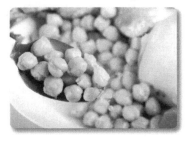

Serves: 1

Calories: 197

Ingredients:

- ½ onion, chopped
- 1 garlic clove, crushed
- 1 tsp olive oil
- ½ red pepper, chopped
- 1 bay leaf
- 250ml/1cup vegetable stock/broth
- ½ tsp mild curry powder
- 15g/ ½ oz long grain or basmati rice
- 1 tsp white wine vinegar
- 40g/ 1 ½ oz small peeled prawns
- 1 tsp tomato puree/paste
- 1 tsp chopped flat leaf parsley

Method:
Dice your potatoes and steam or boil until tender. Drain and leave to cool.

Mix together the paprika, water, cumin, turmeric salt & sugar to form a paste. Add the onion, chickpeas and potatoes to the paste. Combine well and serve with chopped coriander over the top.

Prawn & Rice Soup

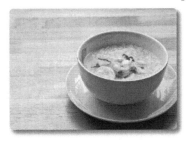

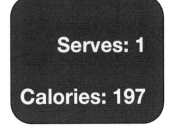

Serves: 1

Calories: 197

Ingredients:

- ½ onion, chopped
- 1 garlic clove, crushed
- 1 tsp olive oil
- ½ red pepper, chopped
- 1 bay leaf
- 250ml/1cup vegetable stock/broth
- ½ tsp mild curry powder
- 15g/ ½ oz long grain or basmati rice
- 1 tsp white wine vinegar
- 40g/ 1 ½ oz small peeled prawns
- 1 tsp tomato puree/paste
- 1 tsp chopped flat leaf parsley

Method:

Gently sauté the onion, garlic and peppers in a heavy pan in the olive oil for a few minutes until soft. Add the curry powder and tomato puree, stir through and add the stock, bay leaf, rice & vinegar. Cover and leave to cook for 10-15 minutes until the rice is tender. Don't stir the soup too much during cooking. Add the prawns and continue to cook until the prawns are pink and piping hot

Mango Melba Salad

Serves: 1

Calories: 199

Ingredients:

- ¼ cantaloupe melon, peeled cubed
- ¼ mango, peeled and cubed
- ½ passion fruit, flesh scooped out and sliced
- 1 tsp olive oil
- ½ tsp cider vinegar
- 25g/ 1oz seedless grapes, halved
- Salt & pepper to taste
- 60ml/ ¼ cup low fat yoghurt
- 1 tsp runny honey
- Pinch ground ginger
- Handful lettuce leaves
- Handful watercress

Method:

Combine the melon, mango and passion fruit with the olive oil and cider vinegar.

Place your lettuce & watercress on a plate and sit the melon mix on top. Mix the honey, yoghurt & ginger together and season. Pour your yoghurt mix over the salad and serve.

Italian Beans

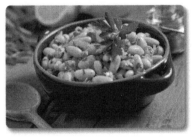 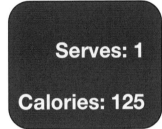

Serves: 1

Calories: 125

Ingredients:

- 100g/3 ½ oz canned cannellini beans
- ½ tsp olive oil
- 1 garlic clove, crushed
- 125ml/ ½ cup vegetable stock/broth

- ½ tsp each dried oregano, basil & thyme
- 1 tbsp lemon juice
- 2 tsp tomato puree/paste
- ½ red onion
- ½ chopped red chilli
- 3 black olives, chopped (optional)

Method:
Gently sauté the onion and garlic in the olive oil. Add all the other ingredients (except olives) and leave to gently cook through for approx. 20 minutes. Add the olives, ensure everything is tender and serve.

Sticky Wings

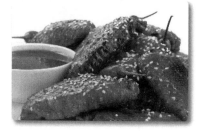

Serves: 1

Calories: 189

Ingredients:

- 2 small chicken wings
- ½ onion finely chopped
- 1 garlic clove, crushed
- 125ml/ ½ cup passata/sieved tomatoes
- 1 tsp each dried thyme & oregano
- 1 tsp Dijon mustard
- 1 tsp brown sugar
- 2 tsp black treacle
- 1 tbsp red wine vinegar
- ¼ tsp salt
- Pinch crushed chilli flakes (or more to taste)
- Low cal spray

Method:

First make the marinade for the chicken by gently frying the onion and garlic in a little low cal spray. Add the passata, herbs, vinegar, sugar, salt, chilli, treacle and mustard. Gently simmer until the sauce has reduced down to about half its original volume. Allow the sauce to cool a little, season well and coat the chicken wings with the sauce. Leave to marinade for an hour or two if possible. Preheat the oven to 220/425/Gas 7, place the chicken and marinade into an oven proof dish and cook for 15-20 mins or until the wings are cooked through.

Spicy Yoghurt Chicken

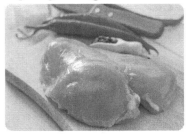

Serves: 1

Calories: 168

Ingredients:

- 1 small skinless chicken breast
- 1 red chilli
- 1 tsp each coriander (cilantro), cumin & turmeric

- ½ each tsp garam masala, paprika & ground ginger
- 1 tbsp lime juice
- 60ml/ ¼ cup low fat yoghurt
- 1 clove garlic, crushed

Method:
Mix the dried spices with the yoghurt. Make some cuts into your chicken breast

And cover with the spicy yoghurt mix. Place under a medium grill and cook for approx. 15 minutes or until properly cooked through.

Thai Mussels

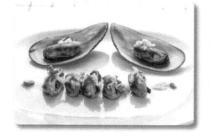

Serves: 1

Calories: 166

Ingredients:

- ½ stalk lemongrass
- 500g/1lb 2oz fresh mussels, cleaned
- 1 tsp fresh coriander/cilantro, chopped
- 2 red or green chillies, sliced
- 1 tsp fish sauce
- ½ tsp sugar
- 2 tsp tamarind paste
- ½ fresh lime
- 2 slices fresh ginger
- 1 tomato, chopped
- Salt & pepper to taste

Method:

Put a pan of 500ml/2 cups salted water on to boil. Add all the ingredients (except lime and fresh coriander) to the pan cover and simmer for 5-6 minutes. Place the cleaned mussels into the pan cover and simmer for a further 6-7 minutes or until the mussels are all open. Discard any that do not fully open. Season and pour the mussel mixture into a bowl. Sprinkle with the coriander and squeeze lime juice over the top.

Marmite Spaghetti

Serves: 1

Calories: 198

Ingredients:

- 75g/3oz spaghetti or linguine
- 7g/ ¼ oz unsalted butter
- ½ tsp Marmite (or jerk sauce)

- Salt & pepper to taste
- 7g/ ¼ oz grated parmesan
- Squirt of ketchup

Method:

Marmite is a real UK specialty, US readers could replace with jerk or hot sauce. Bring a pan of salted water to the boil and cook the spaghetti until tender. While the pasta is cooking, gently heat together the marmite and butter in a large saucepan. When the spaghetti is ready, reserve about a ladle of the pasta water before draining. Add the drained spaghetti to your marmite pan and mix around really well to make sure every strand is covered

If the spaghetti is a little sticky add a splash of your reserved pasta water to loosen it up and divide into bowls. Use squeezy ketchup to make a swirl on the top of your spaghetti and sprinkle with parmesan. Surprisingly delicious.

Eastern Spiced Cod Steak

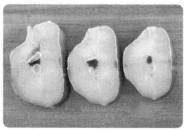

Serves: 1

Calories: 194

Ingredients:

- 140g/5 oz cod steak
- ½ onion
- 1 garlic clove, crushed
- ½ red pepper
- ½ tsp each coriander, cumin, turmeric & garam masala
- 100g/3 ½ oz cherry tomatoes, chopped
- 60ml/ ¼ cup low fat coconut milk
- 1 tsp flat leaf parsley, chopped
- Low cal cooking spray

Method:

Season the fish with salt & pepper. Brown in a frying pan with a little low cal spray for a minute or two each side and remove to a plate. In the same pan, with a little more spray, gently sauté the onion & garlic. Add the spices and cherry tomatoes and get the mixture nice and hot. Place the browned steak on top, cover, reduce the heat and leave to cook for approx. 10 minutes, or until the fish is cooked through. Take the steak out and put on a warm plate. Add the coconut milk to the pan, gently heat and then pour the contents of the pan over the cod. Garnish with the chopped parsley.

Tropical Fruit Salad

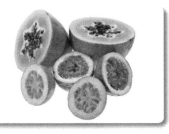

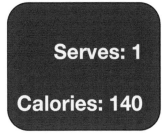

Serves: 1

Calories: 140

Ingredients:

- ¼ papaya (guava),
- ½ banana
- 2 slices of fresh or tinned pineapple

- ½ passion fruit
- 1 tbsp fresh orange

Method:

Peel and slice the banana & cut the pineapple into chunks. Slice the papaya in half and take out the seeds. Scoop out the flesh and slice. Slice the passion fruit in half, scoop out the flesh and slice. Arrange all the fruit into a bowl and pour the orange juice over the top.

Chicken & Corn Skewer

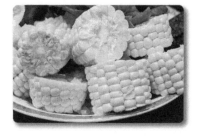

Serves: 1

Calories: 161

Ingredients:

- ½ peeled sweet corn cob cut into 3 slices
- 2 small chicken wings
- 1 wooden skewer

- 2 tbsp lemon juice
- 1 tsp caster/fine sugar
- Salt & pepper to taste

Method:

Brush the chicken and sweet corn with the lemon juice & sugar. Season and spray with a little low cal cooking spray. Skewer a sweet corn slice followed by chicken wing and so on until you have skewered all the chicken and corn in turn. Place under a medium grill and cook for 20 minutes, turning regularly, or until the chicken is cooked through and the sweet corn is tender.

Tomato, Olive & Feta Salad

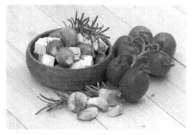

Serves: 1

Calories: 113

Ingredients:

- 2 medium tomatoes sliced
- 1 tsp olive oil
- 25g/1oz reduced fat feta cheese, crumbled

- 1 tsp fresh basil, chopped
- Splash red wine vinegar
- 1 garlic cloves crushed
- 5 pitted olives

Method:
Combine all ingredients together and serve.

Slow Spanish Tombet

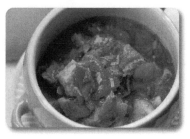

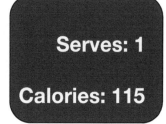

Serves: 1

Calories: 115

Ingredients:

- ½ fresh aubergine/eggplant cubed
- 1 zucchini/courgette, cut into strips
- 1 fresh tomato, cubed
- ¼ red pepper, cut into strips
- 1 tbsp tomato puree/paste
- ½ red onions, sliced

- ½ tsp each of dried marjoram, basil & thyme
- ½ tsp paprika
- ½ tsp capers
- 125ml/ ½ cup water
- Handful pitted black olives
- 1 garlic clove, crushed
- Pinch salt & sugar
- Low cal spray
- Fresh basil to garnish

Method:

Gently sauté the vegetables in the low cal spray, add the herbs, spices and paste. Cook for a further 2 minutes and add the ingredients to the pan. Place on a medium heat on a good simmer and cook until the liquid has reduced to a thick paste and the vegetables are tender.

Sheik Kebab

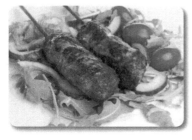

Serves: 1

Calories: 195

Ingredients:

- 75g/3oz lean lamb mince
- ½ tsp ground coriander, garlic, salt
- ½ onion very finely chopped

- 1 green chilli very finely chopped
- ½ tsp mint sauce
- 1 tsp lemon juice
- ½ tsp sunflower oil
- 2 wooden skewers

Method:

Leave 2 wooden skewers to soak in water for a few hours (this prevents them from burning).

Gently fry together the onion, green chillies, coriander (cilantro) and garlic for a few minutes.

Place the lamb, lemon juice and warm spicy onions into a food processor and whizz together until well mixed. Take the mixture out and place on a chopping board. Divide into 4 portions and roll into sausage shapes around each skewer. Grill under a medium heat for 12-15 minutes or until the lamb is properly cooked through.

Bombay Potatoes

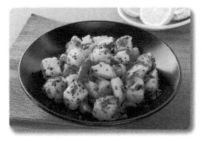

Serves: 1

Calories: 150

Ingredients:

- 1 tsp sunflower oil
- ¼ tsp mustard seeds
- ½ tsp mild chilli powder

- ½ tsp turmeric powder
- 100g potatoes, boiled and cubed
- ½ tsp salt

Method:

Mix the chilli and turmeric in a cup with a little water to form a paste.

Heat the oil in a pan. When it is hot add the mustard seeds and cook for a minute or two until they start to pop. Add the spice paste to the mustard seeds along with the boiled cubed potatoes and cook for a few minutes until the potatoes are completely covered in the spice mix and piping hot.

Latin American Lime Fish

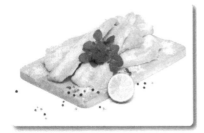

Serves: 1

Calories: 199

Ingredients:

- 100g/3 ½ oz fresh pollock fillets
- 3 tbsp lime juice
- 2 tomatoes, finely chopped
- 1 tbsp fresh coriander/cilantro, chopped
- ½ red onion, sliced into rings
- 3 black olives, finely chopped
- 1 red chilli, finely chopped
- 1 tsp olive oil
- ½ tsp fine caster/fine sugar
- 1 handful fresh watercress

Method:

First slice the pollock into very fine diagonal strips. Mix with the lime juice and sliced red onion. Season well and leave to marinate for at least 40 minutes. The acids of the lime juice will 'cook' the fish.

After this time add all the other ingredients, combine and serve.

Low Fat Hummus & Crackerbread

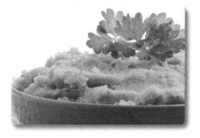

Serves: 1

Calories: 173

Ingredients:

- 100g/3 ½ oz canned chickpeas
- 1 tbsp water
- 1 tsp tahini paste
- ½ garlic clove, chopped
- 1 tbsp low fat Greek yoghurt
- 1 tbsp lemon juice
- Salt & pepper to taste
- 2 wholegrain crackerbread/wheat crackers

Method:

Place all the ingredients in a food processor and pulse until you get a smooth paste. Add a little water to loosen if you need. Adjust your seasoning to taste and serve with crackerbread/wheat crackers.

Baked Brunch For 1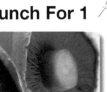

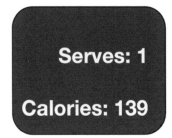

Serves: 1

Calories: 139

Ingredients:

- 1 large flat mushroom
- 2 tomatoes, halved
- ½ garlic clove, crushed

- 50g/2 oz spinach leaves
- 1 free range egg
- Low cal spray
- Salt & pepper

Method:
Preheat your over to 180/350/Gas Mark 6

Take a small oven proof dish and place the halved tomatoes and whole mushroom in. Spray with some low cal spray and season well. Spread the crushed garlic over them.

Throw your spinach into a pan with a tablespoon of water and wilt for a few minutes on a high heat. Add the wilted spinach to your ovenproof dish, make a well in the spinach and crack the egg into the well. Place in the oven and cook for 10 minutes or until the egg is set and the tomatoes are tender

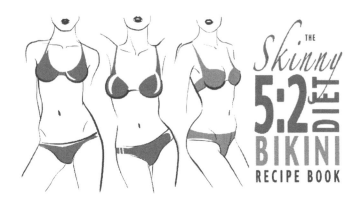

RECIPES UNDER
300 Calories

Spicy Scrambled Egg

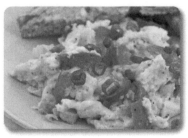

Serves: 1

Calories: 209

Ingredients:

- 2 free range eggs
- 1tsp low fat spread
- ½ red pepper, sliced
- ½ red onion, sliced
- ¼ tsp paprika

- Pinch cayenne pepper
- Salt & pepper to taste

Method:

First gently sauté the pepper and onions in a frying pan using the low cal spread until soft. In a cup, beat your eggs, season and add the paprika and cayenne pepper. Tip the eggs into the pan with the onions and peppers and turn up the heat. Gently mix the eggs constantly until they only just begin to scramble. Remove from heat and serve.

Smoked Salmon On Rye

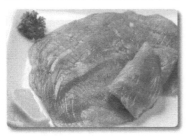

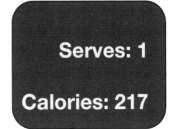

Serves: 1

Calories: 217

Ingredients:

- 75g/3oz smoked salmon slices
- 40g/1 ½ oz radishes, sliced
- 1 tsp poppy seeds
- ½ fresh orange
- ½ tsp cider vinegar
- ½ tsp olive oil
- 2 spring onions/scallions, chopped
- Salt & Pepper to taste
- Rye bread

Method:
Season the smoked salmon with black pepper. Grate the zest from the orange and juice. Combine together the poppy seeds, orange zest and juice, vinegar and olive oil. Add the radishes and spring onions to the bowl and mix. Arrange your salmon slices on your rye bread and pour the radish mixture over the top.

Minted Lamb

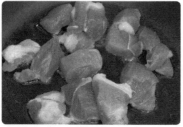

Serves: 1

Calories: 260

Ingredients:

- **75g/3oz lean cubed lamb meat**
- **1 tbsp balsamic vinegar**
- **½ tsp garam masala**
- **½ tsp turmeric**
- **½ tsp garlic**
- **½ tsp coriander (cilantro)**
- **½ tsp salt**
- **½ red onion, chopped**
- **½ tsp mint sauce**
- **1 tsp sunflower oil**
- **60ml/ ¼ cup boiling water**

Method:
Brown the lamb off in a frying pan with the sunflower oil on a high heat. Remove the lamb and very gently fry the onions for a few minutes. Combine the spices and vinegar with the cooking onions, return the meat to the pan and mix well. Add the mixture to an ovenproof dish with the mint sauce and the boiling water (add a little more water if required). Cover and cook in a preheated oven at 180c/350f/gas mark 5 for an hour or until the meat is tender and the water has reduced down.

Aloo Gobi

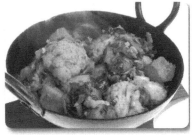

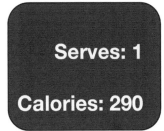

Serves: 1

Calories: 290

Ingredients:

- ½ cauliflower head split into florets
- 200g/7 oz canned chopped tomatoes
- 1 tsp sunflower oil
- ½ onion chopped
- Small handful of shredded green cabbage
- 125g/ 4 ½ oz peeled diced potatoes

- Handful chopped coriander (cilantro)
- ½ tsp chilli powder
- ½ tsp garlic powder
- ½ tsp ground ginger
- ½ tsp sugar
- ½ tsp turmeric
- Pinch cumin
- ½ tsp garam masala
- ½ tsp salt

Method:

Add the oil and onions into a frying pan and gently cook. Mix in the dried herbs, salt and fresh coriander (cilantro) and cook for a further minute or two. Next add the sugar, cabbage, chopped tomatoes, cauliflower and potatoes, cover and cook on the lowest possible setting for at least 20 minutes. Make sure the vegetables are completely tender before serving

Indian Prawns

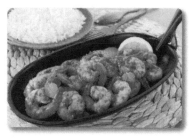

Serves: 1

Calories: 296

Ingredients:

- 200g/7oz small cooked peeled prawns
- 1 tsp sunflower oil
- 1 onions, chopped
- 2 tomatoes, chopped
- ½ red pepper, chopped
- 50g/2oz frozen peas
- ½ tsp each ground cumin, garam masala & coriander (cilantro)
- 1 tbsp lime juice
- ½ tsp salt

Method:
Heat the oil in the pan and gently fry the onion. After a few minutes add the tomatoes, red pepper and peas and leave to cook for about 5 minutes more until the tomatoes start to lose their shape. Add the salt, spices and prawns and cook until the prawns are piping hot. Remove from the heat and stir through the lime juice.

Asian Lentil Salad

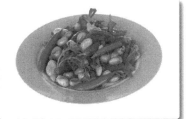

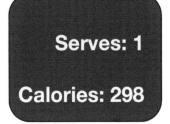

Serves: 1

Calories: 298

Ingredients:

- 40g/1 ½ oz soya beans
- 40g/ 1 ½ oz sugar snap peas
- ½ red chilli, sliced
- 50g/2oz puy lentils
- 250ml/ 1 cup vegetable stock/broth
- 50g/2oz purple sprouting broccoli
- 1 tsp sesame oil
- 1 tsp lemon juice
- ½ garlic clove, crushed
- 1 tbsp soy sauce
- 1 tsp freshly grated ginger
- 1 tsp clear honey
- 2 tbsp water

Method:

Boil the lentils in stock for approx. 10-15 mins until tender. Drain and put in a bowl. In another pan cook the broccoli in a little salted water with the soya beans and sugar snap peas for 2 minutes. Drain and add to the lentils. Mix together the sesame oil, lemon juice, water, garlic, soy sauce, ginger and honey and pour over the top of the lentils and greens.

Trout Fillet & Pine Nuts

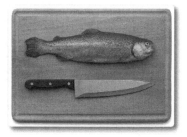 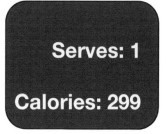

Serves: 1

Calories: 299

Ingredients:

- 115g/4 oz boneless trout fillet
- 15g/ ½ oz breadcrumbs
- 1 tsp low fat spread
- 1 tsp flat leaf parsley, chopped

- 2 tbsp lemon juice
- 7g/ ¼ oz pine nuts, chopped
- 1 tsp olive oil
- 50g/2 oz rocket

Method:
Season the trout. Mix together the breadcrumbs, low fat spread, lemon juice and pine nuts and spread the breadcrumbs mix on top. Place the fillet under a medium grill and cook for approx. 5-10 minutes or until the fish is cooked through. Serve with the rocket on the side.

Turkish Eggs & Peppers

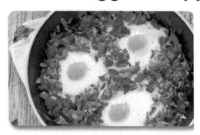

Serves: 1

Calories: 239

Ingredients:

- ½ onion, sliced
- ½ red pepper, sliced
- 1 red chillies, sliced
- 100g/3 ½ oz chopped tomatoes
- ½ tsp paprika
- ½ tsp caster/fine sugar

- 1 egg
- 1 tbsp flat leaf parsley
- 2 tbsp low fat greek yoghurt
- 1 garlic clove, crushed
- Low cal spray

Method:
Heat a little low cal spray in a small frying pan. Sauté the onions, pepper, garlic and chillies for 3-4 minutes. Add the tomatoes and sugar and cook until most of the liquid has reduced. Make a well in the centre of the mixture and crack the egg into it. Season well, cover and leave on a low heat until the egg is set.

Slide onto a plate and serve with yoghurt on the side with the paprika sprinkled over.

Prawns & Peas

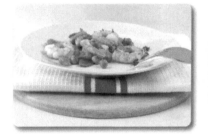

Serves: 1

Calories: 237

Ingredients:

- ½ onion, sliced
- 2 tomatoes, chopped
- 1 tsp freshly grated ginger
- 2 garlic cloves, crushed
- 1 tbsp medium curry powder
- 3 tbsp water
- 100g/3 ½ oz shelled raw king prawns
- 100g/3 ½ oz peas
- 1 tbsp coriander (cilantro), chopped
- Low cal cooking spray

Method:

Heat a little low cal spray in a frying pan, and sauté the onions for a few minutes. Add the garlic and ginger to the onions, cook for a minute longer and add the curry paste and water. Add the peas and chopped tomatoes and cook until the peas are tender. Add the prawns to the mixture and cook until they are bright pink and piping hot throughout. Sprinkle with the chopped coriander (cilantro) and serve.

Special Fried 'Rice'

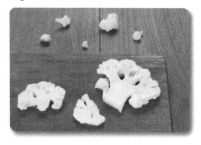

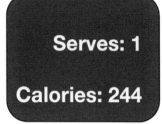

Serves: 1

Calories: 244

Ingredients:

- 1 egg, beaten
- 1 sliced lean back bacon
- 100g/ 3 ½oz mushrooms, sliced
- 100g peas
- 1 garlic clove, crushed

- 1 tsp freshly grated ginger
- 1 tsp soy sauce
- 1 tsp sugar
- ½ head cauliflower
- Low cal spray

Method:
First make your 'rice': take ½ head of cauliflower and whizz in a food processor until you get crumbs the size of rice grains. Cook your peas in a pan of water or the microwave. Heat a little low cal spray in a frying pan, and cook your bacon and mushrooms. Remove from the pan and chop. Add the 'rice' to the pan, stir and add the egg. Keep on stirring and add the egg, bacon, peas and mushrooms to the pan along with the garlic, ginger, soy sauce, & sugar. Cook everything until piping hot. Plate up and serve.

Japanese Beef Salad

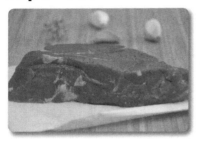

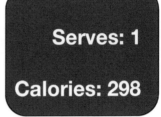

Serves: 1

Calories: 298

Ingredients:

- 125g/4oz fresh sirloin steak,
- 125ml/ ½ cup vegetable stock/broth
- 1 ½ tbsp soy sauce
- 2 ½ tbsp mirin
- ½ tbsp golden caster sugar
- ½ onion, sliced
- 1 tsp chopped pickled ginger
- 1 spring onion/scallion, finely chopped
- ½ red chilli, thinly sliced
- Handful baby spinach

Method:

To start with put the fresh steak in the freezer (this makes it easier to slice). After half an hour take the steak out and slice it as thinly as you possibly can. Mix together the stock, soy, mirin and sugar in a pan and boil. Throw the onions in and cook for 2 minutes, add the sliced beef to the pan and cook for a further 2 minutes until the liquid is reduced and the beef cooked. Place the contents of the pan on a plate on top of the raw spinach leaves and sprinkle with pickled ginger, spring onions and chilli.

Hoisin Chicken Stir Fry

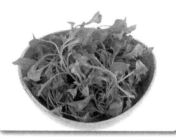

Serves: 1

Calories: 281

Ingredients:

- Low cal cooking spray
- ½ small skinless and boneless chicken breast cut into strips
- 1 red pepper, sliced
- ½ red onion, sliced
- 75g/3oz watercress
- 2 tsp hoisin sauce
- 2 tsp soy sauce
- ½ tsp freshly grated ginger
- 1 garlic clove, crushed
- 1 tsp sesame oil
- 1 tsp white wine vinegar
- 1 tbsp water

Method:
First make a sauce by mixing together the hoisin sauce with the soy sauce, water, ginger, garlic, sesame oil and vinegar. Heat a little low cal oil in a frying pan and cook the chicken, pepper and onions on a high heat for approx. 5 mins until the chicken is cooked. Pour over the sauce, cook for 30 secs, stir through the watercress and serve.

Coconut & Sweet Potato Soup

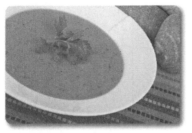

Serves: 1

Calories: 247

Ingredients:

- 1 onion, chopped
- 1 tbsp coconut cream
- 1 tbsp coriander (cilantro), chopped
- 200g/7oz sweet potatoes, grated
- 1 tsp red Thai curry paste, red or green
- 250ml/1 cup vegetable stock/broth

Method:
Sauté the onions in a frying pan with a little low cal cooking spray. After a few minutes stir through the curry paste, grated sweet potato and stock. Cook until tender (about 5-10 minutes) and blend. Add the coconut milk. Season and serve with chopped coriander on top

Thai Mini Chicken Burgers

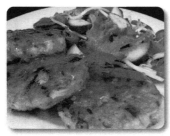

Serves: 1

Calories: 296

Ingredients:

- 1 small skinless chicken breast, chopped
- 1 garlic clove, crushed
- 1 tsp freshly ground ginger
- 1 shallot, chopped
- 1 tbsp fresh coriander
- ½ green chilli
- Low cal spray
- 1 tsp sweet chilli sauce
- 50g/2oz rocket

Method:
Pulse the chicken, garlic, ginger, onion, coriander and chilli in a food processor until everything is breadcrumb size. Season well. Scoop the mix out and shape into 2-3 small patties. Heat a little low cal spray in a frying pan and fry the patties for approx. 8 minutes, or until piping hot and cooked through. Serve with sweet chilli sauce and rocket.

Smoked Salmon & Prawn Salad

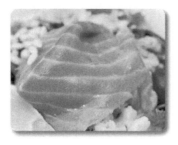

Serves: 1

Calories: 278

Ingredients:

- 1 tbsp lime juice
- ½ tsp runny honey
- Pinch ground ginger
- 75g/3oz salad leaves
- ½ tbsp low fat crème fraiche
- ½ tsp horseradish sauce
- 3 slices smoked salmon
- 6 large cooked king prawns

Method:

Combine the crème fraiche with the horseradish, lime juice, honey, ginger and seasoning. Place your salad leaves on a plate, sit the salmon and prawns on top and cover with the crème fraiche dressing.

Chicken & Haricot Stew

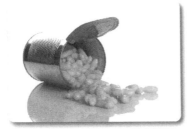

Serves: 1

Calories: 297

Ingredients:

- 100g/ 3 ½ oz boneless, skinless chicken thighs
- 1 onion, finely chopped
- 1 carrot, finely chopped
- 1 celery stick, finely chopped
- ½ tsp dried thyme
- 1 bay leaf
- 180ml/ ¾ cup chicken stock/broth
- 50g /2oz canned haricot beans, drained
- 1 tbsp flat leaf parsley, chopped
- Low cal cooking spray

Method:

Chop up your chicken into chunks. Season and brown in a frying pan with a little low cal oil. Add the onion, carrot & celery and cook for a few minutes. Stir in the herbs and stock, bring up to heat, cover, reduce the heat and leave to simmer for 30mins. Check the chicken is cooked through. Add the haricot beans and cook for a further 4-5 minutes until the beans are piping hot. Serve with parsley sprinkled over the top.

Chicken Noodle Ramen

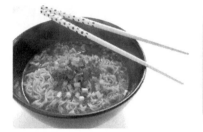

Serves: 1

Calories: 220

Ingredients:

- 100g shirataki noodles
- 1 tbsp sweet corn kernels
- 250ml/1 cup vegetable stock/broth
- 1/2 small skinless chicken breast

- ½ tsp chopped fresh root ginger
- 1 garlic clove, crushed
- 2-3 mushrooms, thinly sliced
- 2 spring onions/scallions, chopped
- 1 tsp soy sauce

Method:

Add the chicken breast piece, stock, ginger and garlic to a pan. Bring to the boil, cover and leave to simmer for 10-15 minutes. Take out the chicken breast and add all the other ingredients to the stock (except spring onions). Simmer for 2-3 minutes until everything is tender. Meanwhile shred your cooked chicken breast and add back into the stock. Pour into a bowl and garnish with your chopped spring onions.

Broccoli & Stilton Soup

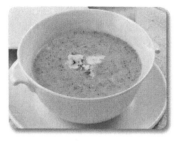

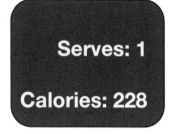

Serves: 1

Calories: 228

Ingredients:

- ½ onion, chopped
- ½ small potato, peeled and cubed
- 250ml/1 cup vegetable stock/broth
- 100g/ 3 ¼ oz broccoli, roughly chopped

- 25g/1oz Stilton cheese, crumbled
- 1 tsp chopped chives
- Low cal cooking spray

Method:

Sauté the onion in a little low cal spray for a few minutes. Add the potato and stock and gently simmer for about 10 mins until the potato is tender. Add the broccoli and cook for another 3 mins. Add the cheese and put the soup in a blender. Season well and serve with chives over the top.

Salmon & Couscous

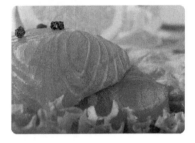

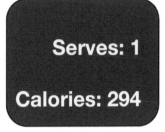

Serves: 1

Calories: 294

Ingredients:

- 40g/ 1 ½ oz couscous
- 1 tsp olive oil
- 140g / 5 oz skinless salmon fillets
- 100g/3 ½ oz purple sprouting broccoli, roughly chopped
- 1 tbsp lemon juice
- 1 large handful watercress
- Olive oil and extra lemon wedges, to serve

Method:
Heat up a pan of water to boiling. Add a pinch of salt. Meanwhile place your couscous in a bowl and pour over boiling water until it just covers the grains. Tip the broccoli into the pan of boiling water, season the salmon and place in the steamer on top of the pan. Cook for approx. 5 mins until the salmon is cooked and the broccoli tender. Drain the broccoli and put to one side with the cooked salmon. Check the couscous is tender, drain the water off and fluff, and toss into a large bowl with the broccoli, olive oil and lemon juice. Season everything well, put your vegetables and couscous on a plate and sit the salmon on top. Serve with wedges of lemon.

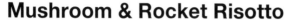

Mushroom & Rocket Risotto

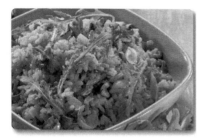

Serves: 1

Calories: 299

Ingredients:

- 1 tsp olive oil
- 100g/3 ½ oz chestnut mushrooms, sliced
- 25g/1oz quinoa
- 250ml/1 cup vegetable stock/broth

- 50g/2oz risotto rice
- 1 tsp dried thyme
- 1 tsp parmesan cheese
- 1 tsp lemon juice
- 25g/1oz rocket
- Salt & pepper to taste

Method:

Gently sauté the mushrooms in the olive oil for a few minutes. Add the quinoa & rice and to coat in the oil. Pour a quarter of your hot stock into the rice mixture and stir until absorbed. Season well, add the thyme and repeat until all your stock is gone and the rice and quinoa are tender and cooked through (add a little more water if needed). When the risotto is ready stir in the rocket, plate up and sprinkle with parmesan and lemon juice.

Spicy Broccoli & Chicken Salad

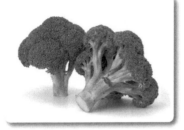

Serves: 1

Calories: 289

Ingredients:

- 1 small chicken breast
- ½ head broccoli, split into florets
- 2 shallots , finely sliced

- 5 pitted black olives, chopped
- 1 tbsp soy sauce
- 1 red chillies, deseeded and sliced
- 1 garlic clove, sliced

Method:
First season and grill the chicken for 10-15 minutes or until cooked through. When it's cooked, rest for a minute or two and slice into diagonal salad size pieces. Meanwhile gently sauté the onion, garlic and olives in a frying pan for a few minutes using a little low cal spray. Steam the broccoli until tender (about 6 mins) and combine in a bowl with the softened onions, garlic, olives and cooked chicken. Arrange on a plate. Add the soy sauce to the now empty frying pan and gently warm through. Pour the warm soy over the plate of salad.

Salmon & Spinach

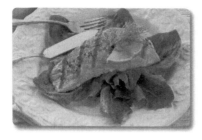

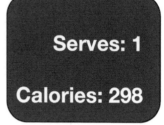

Serves: 1

Calories: 298

Ingredients:

- 140g/ 5 oz skinless salmon fillet
- 125g/4oz baby spinach
- 1 tsp capers, drained and chopped
- 1 tbsp flat leaf parsley, finely chopped
- Lemon wedges to serve
- Salt & pepper to taste
- Pinch crushed chilli flakes (optional)
- Low cal cooking spray

Method:

Put a little low cal spray into a frying pan and place on a medium heat. Season the salmon filet and cook for approx. 3-4 minutes each side or until cooked through (you should be able to flake cooked fix with a fork). Put the fillet on a plate, then transfer your spinach leaves and capers into the frying pan. Season and stir for a minute or two until the leaves wilt. Serve with lemon juice squeezed over the top.

Citrus Ground Lamb

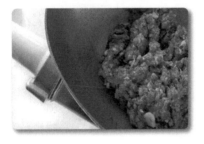

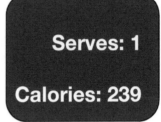

Serves: 1

Calories: 239

Ingredients:

- 100g/3 ½ oz lean minced/ground lamb
- 1 clove garlic, crushed
- ½ tsp ground cumin & coriander
- ½ red onion, sliced

- 1 tsp soy sauce
- 2 tbsp orange juice
- ¼ large fresh orange
- 1 tsp orange zest
- Salt & Pepper to taste

Method:
Brown the mince in a dry frying pan. After a few minutes add all the ingredients (except the fresh orange) to the pan and continue to cook. Cover and leave to simmer for approx. 10 minutes or until the lamb is cooked through. Add a little water during cooking if needed. Meanwhile split your orange into segments, and peel them if you can. When the lamb is ready gently stir though the orange slices and serve.

Simple Sweet & Sour Drummers

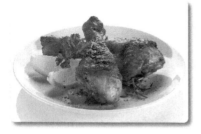

Serves: 1

Calories: 214

Ingredients:

- 2 small chicken drumsticks, skinned
- 1 tbsp red wine vinegar
- 1 tbsp pineapple juice (if you have it)
- ½ tbsp tomato puree/paste
- ½ tbsp. soy sauce
- ½ tsp paprika
- 2 tsp runny honey
- 1 tsp Worcestershire sauce (or jerk sauce)
- ½ Garlic clove, crushed

Method:
First make your sweet and sour sauce; combine the vinegar, soy sauce, tomato puree, Worcestershire sauce, paprika, honey and garlic together in a shallow bowl. Season your chicken and add to the bowl. Cover the chicken in the paste and leave to marinade in the fridge for as long as possible (at least an hour or two ideally). Transfer to an ovenproof dish and grill for approx. 15-20 minutes or until the chicken is cooked through. Keep on turning the chicken throughout cooking to keep them covered with the marinade.

Tuna Potato Salad

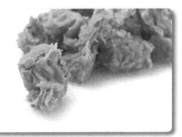

Serves: 1

Calories: 229

Ingredients:

- 100g/3 ½ oz salad potatoes
- ½ pepper sliced, red or green is fine
- 15g/ ½ oz sweet corn kernels
- ½ red onion, chopped
- 75g/3oz tinned tuna steak in spring water
- Handful chopped black olives
- 1 tsp low fat mayonnaise
- 1 tbsp lemon juice
- 1 tsp low fat natural yoghurt
- 1 garlic clove, crushed
- Salt & Pepper to taste

Method:

Boil or steam the salad potatoes until tender. Drain and leave to cool. Mix together the mayonnaise, yoghurt, garlic & lemon juice and season well. Flake the tuna and mix with the cooked salad potatoes, pepper, onion and sweet corn. Add the mayonnaise dressing, combine and sprinkle with the chopped olives.

Steak & Peanut Salad

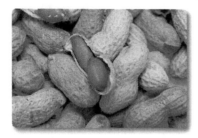

Serves: 1

Calories: 211

Ingredients:

- Handful shredded cabbage
- ½ carrot, peeled and cut into thin batons
- 3 radishes, sliced
- 3 baby sweet corn, halved lengthways
- 100g/ 3 ½ oz sirloin steak

- 1 ½ tsp soy sauce
- ½ tsp groundnut oil
- 15g/ ½ oz plain peanuts, chopped
- ½ red chilli, chopped
- ½ tsp caster sugar
- 1 tsp peanut butter
- Salt & Pepper to taste

Method:
Season your steak and cut into fine strips. Begin stir-frying the steak pieces in the groundnut oil for 3-4 minutes. Add all the other ingredients to the pan (except the chopped peanuts, radishes, carrots and sweet corn) and stir fry briskly for 2 minutes to make sure everything is really well coated. Place the cooked stir fry on a plate, sprinkle with the chopped peanuts and arrange the raw sweet corn, radishes and carrot batons around the dish.

Red Curry Thai Chicken

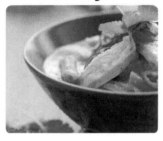

Serves: 1

Calories: 226

Ingredients:

- **1 small skinless chicken breast**
- **125ml/ ½ cup low fat coconut milk**
- **5 cherry tomatoes, halved**
- **½ red pepper, sliced**
- **½ tsp ground ginger**
- **1 tbsp chopped coriander/cilantro**

- **1 clove garlic, crushed**
- **½ tbsp Thai red curry paste**
- **50g/2oz sweet potato, peeled and cut into small batons**
- **Low cal cooking spray**

Method:
Slice your chicken breast. Season and stir fry in a little low cal cooking spray. Add the tomatoes, pepper, ginger, garlic and curry paste and cook for 2 minutes. Add the coconut milk and very gently simmer for 15 mins, or until the chicken is cooked and the sweet potato is tender. Sprinkle with chopped coriander and serve.

Pork & Apple Medallions

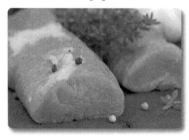

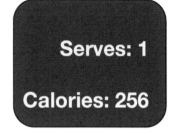

Serves: 1

Calories: 256

Ingredients:

- 2 x pork tenderloin medallions (approx. 100g)
- ½ red onion
- ½ clove garlic, crushed
- ½ tsp caster/fine sugar
- ½ tsp dried sage
- 60ml/ ¼ cup dry cider
- 60ml/ ¼ cup vegetable stock/broth
- 1 apple, cored and sliced
- 1 tsp lemon juice
- Low cal cooking spray

Method:
Gently sauté the onions and garlic in a little low cal spray. Add the sugar and stir well. Place the pork in the pan and cook for 3-4 minutes until browned. Add all the ingredients (except the apple slices & lemon) to the pan and leave to simmer for approx. 15-20 minutes or until the liquid is reduced to almost nothing. Mix the apple slices with the lemon juice and add to the pan, continue to cook for a minute or two longer.

Plaice & Mixed Mushrooms

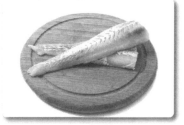

Serves: 1

Calories: 243

Ingredients:

- 125g/ 4 ½ oz boneless plaice fillet
- 2 cloves garlic, crushed
- ¼ tsp salt
- ¼ tsp onion powder
- 2 tsp lemon juice
- 100g/3 ½ oz mixed mushrooms (use whichever varieties you prefer)
- 1 fresh tomato, chopped
- 1 tbsp chopped fresh basil
- Low cal spray

Method:

Mix together the garlic, salt, onion powder & lemon juice and brush the fish fillet with the mixture. Grill under a medium heat for 8-10 minutes. In the meantime gently sauté the tomatoes, mushrooms and basil in a little low cal spray for a few minutes until the mushrooms are cooked through. Serve on top of the plaice fillet.

The Best Mussels

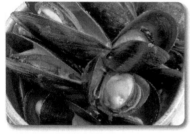

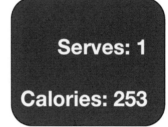

Serves: 1

Calories: 253

Ingredients:

- 1 tsp olive oil
- ½ onion, chopped
- 1 garlic clove, crushed
- 1 tsp rosemary, finely chopped
- 1 bay leaf
- 100g/3 ½ oz chopped tomatoes
- ½ tsp caster sugar
- ¼ tsp salt
- 60ml/ ¼ cup dry white wine
- 2 tsp tomato puree/paste
- 4 chopped olives
- 175g/6oz fresh mussels
- 1 tbsp flat leaf parsley, chopped

Method:
Gently sauté the olives, onion, garlic, tomatoes, sugar, salt, rosemary, garlic for a few minutes. Add the puree & wine and season. Leave to simmer for 10 minutes. Meanwhile place your mussels into a pan with a little boiling water in the base. Cover and leave the mussels on a high heat to steam for a few minutes until they open up. Throw away any that do not open. Place the cooked mussels in a bowl and spoon over your tomato sauce and sprinkle over the parsley. Delicious.

Aromatic Tuna Steaks

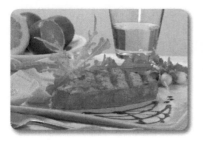

Serves: 1

Calories: 239

Ingredients:

- **175g/6oz fresh tuna steak**
- **½ tsp olive oil**
- **½ clove garlic, crushed**
- **Pinch each of ground cumin, coriander (cilantro) & paprika**

- **1 tsp lime juice**
- **1 tsp coriander (cilantro) freshly chopped**
- **Salt & Pepper to taste**

Method:
Mix together the garlic, oil, dried spices, salt & pepper to make a paste.

Season the tuna steak well and brush the paste onto both sides of the steak.

Put a dry frying pan onto a medium/high heat, when it's good and hot place the tuna steak in the pan and cook for 2-4 minutes each side (depending on how well cooked you like your tuna). Sprinkle with the lime juice and chopped coriander before serving.

Spicy Lamb Fillet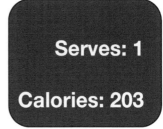

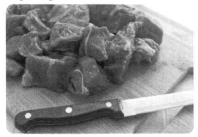

Serves: 1

Calories: 203

Ingredients:

- 75g/3oz Lean Lamb Fillet
- 1 tsp olive oil
- 2 tsp horseradish sauce
- 2 tsp plain/all purpose flour

- 2 tsp brown sugar
- 2 tsp wholegrain mustard
- Salt & Pepper to taste

Method:
Preheat the oven to 200 C / 400 F / Gas Mark 5

Combine the oil, sugar, mustard, horseradish sauce and flour into a bowl. Season your lamb fillet and cover in the flour mixture by rolling the fillet in the bowl.

Loosely wrap the lamb in foil in a 'tent' which will keep all the heat and juices in. Place in the oven and cook for 20-30 mins or until the lamb is tender and cooked to your taste. When the lamb is ready rest for a few minutes and then slice into diagonal strips. Pour any left over foil juices over the top of the meat.

Mexican Chicken

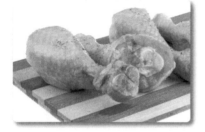

Serves: 1

Calories: 207

Ingredients:

- Low cal cooking spray
- 2 small chicken drumsticks
- ½ onion, chopped
- ½ tsp each ground coriander
- 1 tsp tomato puree/paste
- 40g/ 1 ½ oz sweet corn kernels
- 125g/4oz tinned chopped tomatoes
- Pinch cayenne pepper (or more to taste)
- Salt & Pepper to taste

Method:

Season the chicken, spray a frying pan with a little low cal oil and brown the chicken all over. Add the onion, coriander and cayenne pepper and sauté for a few minutes. Combine the rest of the ingredients in the pan, stir well, cover and leave to gently simmer for approx. 20 minutes or until the chicken is cooked through. Add a little water during cooking if need be.

Cooked Breakfast Muffin

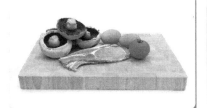

Serves: 1

Calories: 210

Ingredients:

- ½ wholemeal muffin
- 1 slice lean bacon
- 1 egg
- 1 tomato
- 1 large flat mushroom
- 1 tsp fresh chives
- Low cal cooking spray
- Salt & pepper to taste

Method:

Spray the tomato & mushroom with low cal spray, season well, and place under a preheated grill. After a few minutes of cooking place the bacon under the grill too. Meanwhile poach your egg and toast your muffin. When everything is ready pile on top of the muffin and sprinkle with chopped chives.

Chicken Focaccia

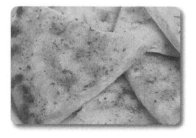

Serves: 1

Calories: 245

Ingredients:

- ½ small skinless chicken breast
- ¼ red onion, left whole
- ¼ avocado, flesh stopped out
- 2 tsp lemon juice
- 2 tsp low fay mayonnaise
- 1 fresh tomato, cut into 4 wedges
- Pinch cayenne pepper (or more to taste)
- 1 slice low fat focaccia bread (no more than 85 cals)
- 50g green salad leaves
- Low cal cooking oil
- Salt & Pepper to taste

Method:

Season your chicken, onion & tomato and spray with low cal cooking oil. Grill under a medium heat until the chicken is cooked through and the tomato & onion chargrilled (remove earlier than chicken if already cooked). Meanwhile mash together the scooped out avocado flesh and lemon with a fork, season and sprinkle the cayenne pepper on top. When the chicken is cooked slice in diagonal strips. Combine with avocado mash and place on top of the focaccia along with the tomato and onion. Serve with salad on the side.

Shami Tikka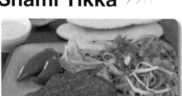

Serves: 1

Calories: 210

Ingredients:

- 75g/3oz lean lamb mince
- ½ tsp ground coriander (cilantro), garlic, salt, paprika, cumin & turmeric
- ½ onion very finely chopped
- ½ green chilli very finely chopped
- 1 tsp freshly chopped mint
- 1 tsp lemon juice
- 1 tbsp low fat yoghurt
- Pinch paprika
- Low cal spray

Method:

Gently fry together the onion, green chillies, coriander (cilantro), paprika, cumin, turmeric and garlic in a little low cal spray for a few minutes.

Place the lamb, lemon juice, chopped mint and warm spicy onions into a food processor and whizz together until well mixed. Take the mixture out and place on a chopping board. Divide into 4 portions and shape into small flat meat patties. Grill under a medium heat for 10-12 minutes or until the lamb is properly cooked through.

Serve with the lettuce and low fat yoghurt with the paprika sprinkled on the top.

Lime & Chilli Mackerel

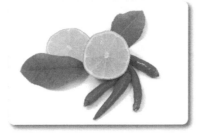

Serves: 1

Calories: 282

Ingredients:

- 1 small whole fresh mackerel, gutted (125 g/ 4 ½ oz)
- ½ clove garlic, crushed
- ¼ tsp each ground cumin, coriander & paprika
- 1 tbsp chopped coriander (cilantro)
- 1 red chilli, deseeded and finely chopped
- 1 tsp olive oil
- 1 fresh lime
- Salt & pepper to taste

Method:

Mix together the dry spices, chilli, garlic and olive oil. Brush the fish all over with the oil mixture and season with salt & pepper. Place under a medium grill and cook for 4-5 minutes each side or until cooked through. Squeeze lime juice over the top and serve with a lime wedge.

Pasta Carbonara

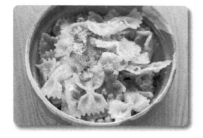

Serves: 1

Calories: 294

Ingredients:

- 75g/3oz pasta
- 50ml low fat crème fraiche
- ½ egg (break an egg into a bowl and beat so you can pour half out)

- 25g/1oz frozen peas
- ½ slice lean bacon
- 7g ¼ oz parmesan cheese

Method:

Cook your pasta and bacon separately. When the bacon is crisp chop into small pieces, meanwhile cook the peas (you can throw them in with the pasta for the last 6-7 minutes of cooking). Drain and put the pasta and peas back into the pan. Beat together the crème fraiche and egg and add to the pan along with the bacon. Put back on a very low heat and stir until warmed through, but don't turn the sauce into scrambled egg!

Sprinkle with parmesan and serve immediately

Chicken Tikka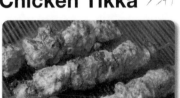

Serves: 1

Calories: 240

Ingredients:

- 1 small skinless chicken breast
- 75g/3oz low fat natural yoghurt
- ½ tsp each turmeric ground cumin, garam masala, coriander, mild chilli powder, garlic powder
- 2 cherry tomatoes
- ¼ tsp ground ginger
- 1 tsp lemon juice
- Pinch salt

Method:
Mix all the spices and lemon juice and a drop of water together to form a paste.

Add yoghurt and mix through. Combine the meat into the mixture and leave to marinade in the fridge overnight.

Put the meat pieces on wooden skewers with the tomatoes and cook in a pre-heated oven at 200C/400F/Gas Mark 6 for approx. 15 minutes or until the meat is properly cooked through.

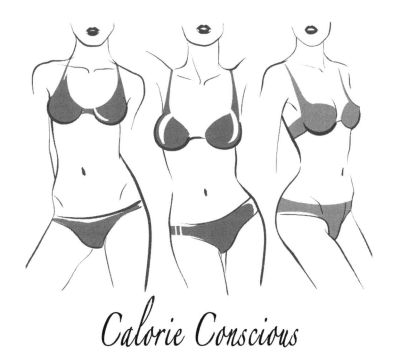

Calorie Conscious

Calorie Conscious

There is endless calorie information available for free online. It's almost impossible to put together a comprehensive resource as part of a book and so the list here is intended as nothing more than a guide to some of the more popular fruit, salad & vegetables to help you get a handle on food calories. All food calories are listed per 100g of the stated food.

Per 100g/3 ½ oz

Vegetables & Salad

Asparagus	20 cals
Beansprouts	30 cals
Broccoli	34 cals
Brussel Sprouts	42 cals
Butternut Squash	45 cals
Carrots	41 cals
Cauliflower	25 cals
Celery	14 cals
Courgette/ Zucchini	16 cals
Cucumber	15 cals
Frozen Peas	64 cals
Green Peas	81 cals
Green Pepper	20 cals
Leeks	61 cals
Mixed Salad	17 cals
Mushrooms	22 cals
Pak Choi	13 cals
Parsnips	67 cals
Potatoes	75 cals
Red Cabbage	31 cals
Savoy Cabbage	27 cals
Spinach	23 cals
Sweet Potato	86 cals
Sweetcorn	86 cals
Tomatoes	18 cals
Wild Rocket	17 cals

Fruit (per 100g/3 ½ oz)

Apples	52 cals
Avacado	160 cals
Banana	89 cals
Blackberries	43 cals
Blueberries	57 cals
Cantaloupe Melon	34 cals
Cherries	63 cals
Grapefruit	32 cals
Grapes	69 cals
Kiwi	61 cals
Oranges	47 cals
Peached canned	44 cals
Peaches	39 cals
Pears	58 cals
Pineapple	48 cals
Plums	46 cals
Raspberries	52 cals
Strawberries	32 cals
Watermelon	30 cals

Other CookNation Titles

You may also be interested in other titles in the CookNation series:

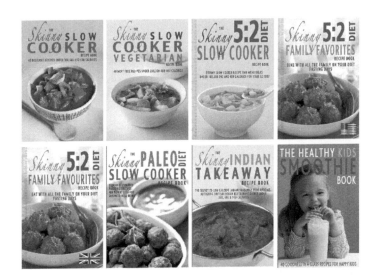

The Skinny 5:2 Slow Cooker Recipe Book
Skinny Slow Cooker Recipe And Menu Ideas Under 100, 200, 300 & 400 Calories For Your 5:2 Diet.

The Skinny 5:2 Family Favourites Recipe Book
(UK & US Editions)
Eat With All the Family On Your Diet Fasting Days.

The Skinny Slow Cooker Recipe Book
40 Delicious Recipes Under 300, 400 And 500 Calories

The Skinny Slow Cooker Vegetarian Recipe Book
40 Delicious Recipes Under 200, 300 And 400 Calories
The Skinny Paleo Diet Slow Cooker Recipe Book
Over 40 Gluten Free Paleo Diet Recipes For Weight Loss And Enhanced Well Being

The Skinny Indian Takeaway Recipe Book
Authentic British Indian Restaurant Dishes Under 300, 400
And 500 Calories

The Healthy Kids Smoothie Book
40 Delicious Goodness In A Glass Recipes for Happy Kids

Find all these great titles by searching under **'CookNation'**
on Amazon.